The Ultimate GERD Diet Plan

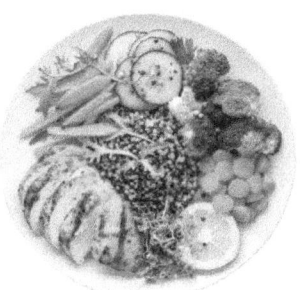

Delicious Recipes and a 30-Day
Meal Guide to Relieve
Heartburn, Acid Reflux, and
Restore Gut Health

Lisa Sharon

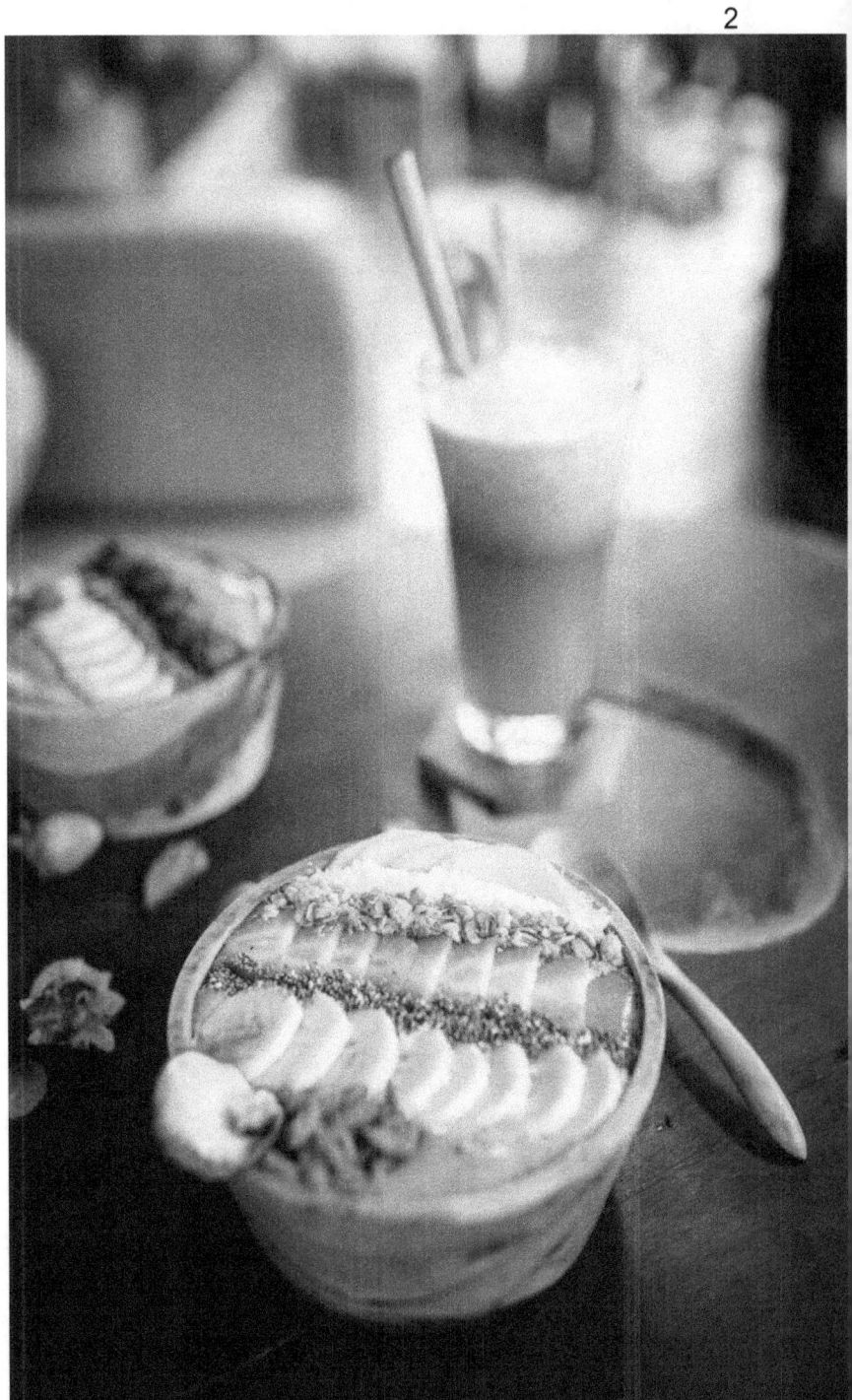

Healthy Diet

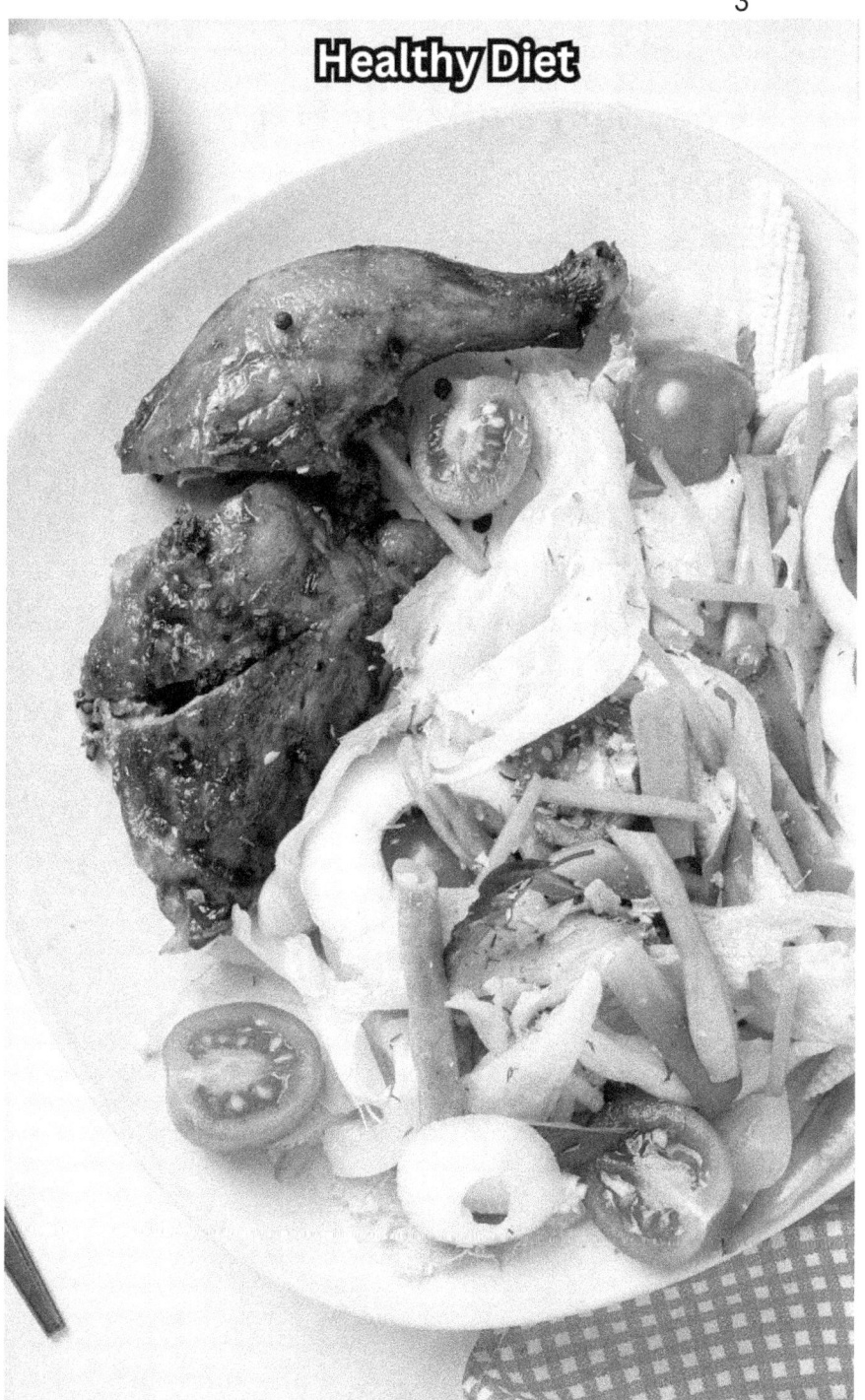

Table Of Contents

Introduction. 9

Understanding GERD .. **Error! Bookmark not defined.**

Causes, Symptoms, and Impact on Digestive Health........... **Error! Bookmark not defined.**

The Role of Diet in Managing GERD .... **Error! Bookmark not defined.**

Chapter 1 15

Foods to Embrace 15

Low-Acid Fruits and Vegetables 16

Whole Grains and Lean Proteins 19

Healthy Fats and Probiotics 20

Chapter 2 24

Foods to Avoid 24

Acidic and Spicy Foods 24

The Hidden Triggers 24

Fried and Fatty Foods 26

The Heavy Hitters 26

Caffeinated and Carbonated Beverages 27

The Bubbly Troublemakers.................. 27

Smart Substitutions for Common Triggers 28

Timing Matters.................................... 29

Beyond What You Eat 29

Listen to Your Body 30

Chapter 3 31

Meal Planning for GERD 31

Your Blueprint for Balanced, Comfortable Eating 31

Developing a Balanced GERD-Friendly Diet 32

The Foundation of Balance 32

Building Blocks of a GERD-Friendly Diet 33

Portion Control and Pacing Meals 34

The Art of Portion Control 34

Meal Timing and Frequency 34

Incorporating Fiber and Hydration 36

Smart Hydration Strategies 37

Practical Meal Planning Tips 37

Creating Balanced Meals 38

Success Strategies 39

Chapter 4 41

Breakfast Favorites 41

Start Your Day with Joy, Not Heartburn 41

The Magic of Morning Meals 42

Prep-Ahead Secrets 50

Chapter 5 52

Lunchtime Solutions 52

Your Midday Menu for Happy Digestion ... 52

Power-Packed Lunches That Love You Back 53

Lunch Success Strategies 60

Packing for Work or Travel 61
Mix and Match Components 61
Chapter 6 64
Delightful Dinners 64
Ending Your Day on a Happy, Heartburn-Free Note 64
The Secret to GERD-Friendly Evening Meals 65
Evening Meal Success Strategies 72
Make-Ahead Tips for Busy Days 73
Quick Substitutions 73
Chapter 7 75
Snacks and Sides 75
Your Go-To Guide for Happy Snacking 75
Smart Snacking Strategies 75
Smart Snacking Guidelines 80
Additional Quick Snack Ideas 81
Travel-Friendly Options 82
Emergency Snack Kit 82
Creating Your Perfect Snack Formula 83
Chapter 8 86
Soothing Smoothies and Juices 86
Mango Ginger Smoothie 86
Kale and Apple Green Juice 87
Aloe Vera and Pineapple Refresher ... 88
Chapter 9 91
A 30-Day GERD-Friendly Meal Plan 91
Weekly Meal Schedules 91

Grocery Lists and Preparation Tips 95
Customizable for Individual Dietary
Needs 96
Conclusion 98
A Path to Lasting Relief and Wellness 98
Additional Resources and Support 99

Introduction

Have you ever found yourself lying awake at night, propped up on multiple pillows, wondering if you'll ever enjoy a meal without fear again? If you're holding this book, chances are you know exactly what I'm talking about. Living with **GERD** isn't just about occasional heartburn — **it's about planning your entire life around your digestive system**, and I understand how exhausting that can be.

I'm here to tell you something important: **your journey to better digestive health starts today.** Whether you're newly diagnosed with GERD, have been struggling silently for years, or are searching for answers to help a loved one, you've found your roadmap to relief. This book isn't just another collection of recipes – it's your companion in reclaiming the joy of eating and living well.

Understanding GERD

Causes, Symptoms, and Impact on Digestive Health

Let's be honest – GERD can feel like your body has turned against you. That burning sensation in your chest, the bitter taste in your throat, the constant worry about what foods might trigger your next flare-up – it's all connected to a complex interplay between your digestive system and your lifestyle choices. But here's the good news: understanding your condition is the first step toward managing it effectively.

Think of your digestive system as a carefully orchestrated dance. When GERD disrupts this dance, it's not just about acid reflux – it affects your sleep, your work, your social life, and even your emotional wellbeing. Throughout these pages, we'll break down the science into practical, actionable insights that will help you understand exactly what's happening in your body and why certain changes can make a dramatic difference.

The Role of Diet in Managing GERD

Here's where hope begins to take root. Your diet isn't just about avoiding triggers – it's about embracing foods that can actually help heal and protect your digestive system. Through years of research and working with countless patients, I've discovered that the right dietary approach can transform GERD from a daily struggle into a manageable condition.

In the coming chapters, you'll discover not just what to eat, but why certain foods work for or against you. We'll explore delicious recipes that prove "GERD-friendly" doesn't mean "flavor-free." From quick breakfasts that won't slow you down to family-friendly dinners everyone will love, each recipe has been carefully crafted to nourish your body while respecting its needs.

This isn't about temporary fixes or bland, restrictive diets. This is about creating a sustainable, enjoyable way of eating that fits your real life. Whether you're a busy professional, a parent juggling family meals, or someone who simply wants to enjoy food again without fear, you'll find practical solutions and encouragement in these pages.

Remember, you're not alone in this journey. Millions of people face the challenges of GERD every day, but with the right knowledge and tools, you can take control of your digestive health. Let's turn the page together and start your path to feeling better, one delicious meal at a time.

The solutions you're looking for are right here. Ready to begin?

Chapter 1

Foods to Embrace

Congratulations on taking the first step towards managing your GERD symptoms through the power of food! In this comprehensive chapter, we'll explore the key food groups that should become the cornerstone of your GERD-friendly diet. By incorporating these nourishing, low-irritant ingredients into your meals, you'll be well on your way to finding lasting relief and restoring your digestive health.

Low-Acid Fruits and Vegetables

When it comes to GERD, the acidity level of the foods you consume plays a crucial role. Highly acidic foods, such as citrus fruits, tomatoes, and certain vegetables, can trigger or exacerbate your reflux episodes. Instead, focus on incorporating low-acid produce items that are gentle on the digestive system and can even help soothe irritation in the esophagus.

Start your day with a delicious smoothie made with ripe bananas, which are naturally low in acid and rich in fiber, potassium, and other essential nutrients. Bananas can help neutralize stomach acid and coat the esophageal lining, providing relief from heartburn. Pair your banana smoothie with a side of melon, which is another excellent low-acid fruit option that's hydrating and packed with vitamins and minerals.

Leafy greens, such as spinach, kale, and arugula, are also fantastic GERD-friendly choices. These nutrient-dense veggies are not only low in acidity, but they're also high in antioxidants, which can help reduce inflammation in the digestive tract. Try incorporating them into salads, omelets, or sautéed dishes for a nourishing and reflux-friendly meal.

Broccoli is another superstar vegetable that should be a staple in your GERD-friendly diet. Not only is it low in acid, but it's also a rich source of fiber, which can help regulate digestion and promote feelings of fullness. Roast broccoli florets with a drizzle of olive oil and a sprinkle of sea salt for a delicious and easy side dish.

Whole Grains and Lean Proteins

Whole grains, such as quinoa, brown rice, and oats, are excellent sources of complex carbohydrates that can help stabilize blood sugar levels and promote feelings of fullness. These nutrient-dense grains are also gentle on the digestive system, making them a great choice for individuals with GERD.

When pairing your whole grains, opt for lean protein sources, such as grilled chicken, turkey, or fish. These protein-rich options are easy to digest and won't exacerbate your reflux symptoms. For a well-balanced meal, try a quinoa and vegetable stir-fry with grilled salmon, or a brown rice bowl topped with roasted turkey and sautéed greens.

Healthy Fats and Probiotics

Contrary to popular belief, not all fats are off-limits for individuals with GERD. In fact, incorporating healthy unsaturated fats, like those found in avocados, nuts, seeds, and olive oil, can actually help reduce inflammation and support overall gut health.

Avocados, for example, are a fantastic source of monounsaturated fats, which can help soothe the esophageal lining and reduce the risk of reflux. Sprinkle some diced avocado onto your salads or enjoy it as a creamy topping on whole grain toast. Nuts and seeds, such as almonds, walnuts, and chia seeds, are also great sources of healthy fats and can be enjoyed as snacks or incorporated into your meals.

In addition to healthy fats, probiotic-rich foods can also play a crucial role in managing GERD symptoms. Probiotics, which are the beneficial bacteria that reside in your gut, can help restore the balance of your gut microbiome, reducing inflammation and promoting overall digestive health. Incorporate probiotic-rich foods, such as yogurt, kefir, and fermented vegetables, into your diet to support your gut healing and GERD management.

As you begin to incorporate these GERD-friendly foods into your diet, you'll start to notice a difference in how you feel. Your meals will not only be more enjoyable, but they'll also provide the nourishment your body needs to heal and thrive. Remember, every person's digestive system is unique, so be patient and experiment to find the right balance of foods that work best for you.

Stay tuned for the next chapter, where we'll explore the foods you should aim to limit or avoid in your GERD management plan. Together, we'll create a customized approach that will have you feeling your best in no time.

Chapter 2

Foods to Avoid

Living with GERD doesn't mean you have to give up all your favorite foods forever. However, understanding which foods can trigger symptoms is crucial for managing your condition effectively. In this chapter, we'll explore the foods and beverages that commonly trigger GERD symptoms, helping you make informed choices about your diet.

Acidic and Spicy Foods

The Hidden Triggers

When you're dealing with GERD, certain acidic and spicy foods can be your digestive system's worst enemies. Here's what you need to know:

High-Acid Foods to Limit:

Citrus fruits and juices (oranges, lemons, limes, grapefruit)

Tomatoes and tomato-based products

Vinegar-based dressings and marinades

Pickled or fermented foods

Raw onions and garlic

Why These Foods Matter: These foods can increase stomach acid production and relax the lower esophageal sphincter (LES), the muscle that prevents stomach acid from flowing back into your esophagus. When you consume them, especially on an empty stomach, they can irritate your esophagus and intensify GERD symptoms.

Spicy Foods to Watch:

Hot peppers (jalapeños, habaneros, cayenne)

Hot sauces and pepper-based condiments

Curry dishes with high spice content
Black pepper in large amounts

Pro Tip: If you love spicy foods, try gradually reducing the heat level in your dishes rather than eliminating spice altogether. Many people find they can tolerate mild spices when combined with GERD-friendly foods.

Fried and Fatty Foods

The Heavy Hitters

Fat takes longer to digest, which means it stays in your stomach longer and increases pressure on your LES. Here's what to minimize:

High-Fat Foods to Limit:
Deep-fried foods of any kind
Fatty cuts of meat (bacon, sausage, marbled steaks)
Full-fat dairy products

Creamy sauces and dressings
Butter and margarine in large amounts
Greasy fast food items

Understanding the Impact: These foods not only slow digestion but also require more stomach acid for breakdown. This combination creates the perfect storm for acid reflux episodes.

Caffeinated and Carbonated Beverages

The Bubbly Troublemakers

What you drink can be just as important as what you eat when managing GERD. Here are the beverages to approach with caution:

Caffeinated Drinks to Limit:

Coffee (both regular and decaf can trigger symptoms)
Black tea
Energy drinks

Chocolate drinks

Some sodas

Carbonated Beverages to Watch:

All types of sodas

Sparkling water

Carbonated energy drinks

Beer and sparkling wines

Why These Matter: Both caffeine and carbonation can relax the LES and increase stomach acid production. The bubbles in carbonated drinks can also cause your stomach to expand, putting extra pressure on the LES.

Smart Substitutions for Common Triggers

Instead of feeling deprived, focus on finding satisfying alternatives:

Replace citrus fruits with melons or bananas

Swap coffee for herbal tea (chamomile, licorice, or slippery elm)

Choose baked or grilled options instead of fried foods

Opt for still water with a splash of non-citrus fruit

Timing Matters

Beyond What You Eat

Remember that when you eat is often as important as what you eat. Consider these timing tips:

Avoid eating within 3 hours of bedtime

Space out your meals throughout the day

Eat slowly and mindfully

Keep portions moderate to avoid overfilling your stomach

Listen to Your Body

While these guidelines are helpful, everyone's triggers can be different. Keep a food diary to identify your personal trigger foods. Note not just what you eat, but also:

Time of day

Portion sizes

Combinations of foods

Stress levels

Sleep quality

This information will help you develop a personalized approach to managing your GERD through diet.

Chapter 3

Meal Planning for GERD

Your Blueprint for Balanced, Comfortable Eating

Living with GERD doesn't mean you have to sacrifice enjoyable meals. The key lies in thoughtful planning and understanding how to structure your daily diet. In this chapter, we'll explore how to create satisfying meals that won't trigger your symptoms.

Developing a Balanced GERD-Friendly Diet

The Foundation of Balance

Creating a GERD-friendly diet isn't just about avoiding trigger foods—it's about building a sustainable eating pattern that nourishes your body while keeping symptoms at bay. Here's how to achieve this balance:

The Ideal Plate Method

Structure your main meals using this simple approach:

1/2 plate: Non-acidic vegetables (steamed, roasted, or raw)

1/4 plate: Lean proteins (grilled, baked, or poached)

1/4 plate: Complex carbohydrates (whole grains, sweet potatoes)

Pro Tip: Think of your plate as a canvas where colors and textures work together. The more varied your choices within safe foods, the more nutrients you'll get.

Building Blocks of a GERD-Friendly Diet

1. Proteins

Choose: Skinless chicken, turkey, fish, tofu

Prepare: Grilled, baked, or poached

Portion: 4-6 ounces per meal (about the size of your palm)

2. Complex Carbohydrates

Choose: Brown rice, quinoa, oats, sweet potatoes

Prepare: Well-cooked, never al dente

Portion: 1/2 to 1 cup cooked per meal

3. Vegetables

Choose: Green beans, carrots, broccoli (well-cooked)

Prepare: Steamed until tender

Portion: Fill half your plate

Portion Control and Pacing Meals

The Art of Portion Control

Overeating is one of the main triggers for GERD symptoms. Here's your guide to proper portioning:

Visual Portion Guide

Protein: Palm of your hand

Grains: Cupped hand

Vegetables: Two fists

Healthy fats: Thumb tip

Meal Timing and Frequency

Structure your eating schedule to minimize reflux:

Eat 5-6 smaller meals instead of 3 large ones

Space meals 2-3 hours apart

Last meal should be 3 hours before bedtime

Sample Meal Schedule:
7:00 AM - Breakfast
10:00 AM - Morning snack
12:30 PM - Lunch
3:30 PM - Afternoon snack
6:00 PM - Dinner
(Optional) 7:00 PM - Light snack if needed

Mindful Eating Practices
1. Take Your Time
   Chew thoroughly (aim for 20-30 chews per bite)
   Put utensils down between bites
   Take 20-30 minutes for each meal

2. Create a Calm Environment
   Sit at a table
   Remove distractions
   Focus on your food

Incorporating Fiber and Hydration

The Fiber Factor

Fiber plays a crucial role in digestive health and can help manage GERD symptoms when incorporated properly.

Daily Fiber Goals:
Women: 25 grams
Men: 38 grams

Important: Increase fiber gradually to avoid digestive discomfort.

Best Sources of GERD-Friendly Fiber:
Oatmeal: 4g per cup
Quinoa: 5g per cup
Sweet potatoes: 4g per medium potato
Green beans: 4g per cup
Carrots: 3g per cup

Smart Hydration Strategies

Proper hydration supports digestion but how you hydrate matters.

Hydration Guidelines:

Aim for 8-10 cups of water daily

Sip slowly throughout the day

Avoid large amounts of liquid with meals

Stop drinking 30 minutes before meals

Best Practices:

Keep a water bottle handy

Set reminders to drink regularly

Monitor urine color (pale yellow is ideal)

Practical Meal Planning Tips

Weekly Preparation

1. Plan Your Menu

Write out meals for the week

Create a shopping list

Prep ingredients in advance

2. Batch Cooking

Prepare basic ingredients

Store properly portioned meals

Keep emergency GERD-friendly snacks handy

Creating Balanced Meals

Sample Day Plan:

Breakfast (7:00 AM)

Oatmeal with sliced banana

Handful of almonds

Non-caffeinated herbal tea

Morning Snack (10:00 AM)

Rice cake with almond butter

Small pear

Lunch (12:30 PM)

Grilled chicken breast

Steamed brown rice

Roasted vegetables

Afternoon Snack (3:30 PM)
Carrot sticks with hummus
Small handful of pumpkin seeds

Dinner (6:00 PM)
Baked fish
Quinoa
Steamed green beans
Small side salad with GERD-friendly dressing

Success Strategies

1. Keep a Food Journal
    Track meals and symptoms
    Note portion sizes
    Record timing of meals

2. Plan for Challenges
    Restaurant strategies
    Travel tips
    Social event planning

3. Listen to Your Body

Pay attention to fullness cues

Notice what combinations work best

Adjust portions based on activity level

Remember, successful meal planning with GERD is about creating a sustainable routine that works for your lifestyle while keeping symptoms under control. Start with these guidelines and adjust them to fit your personal needs and preferences.

Chapter 4

Breakfast Favorites

Start Your Day with Joy, Not Heartburn

Hey there, breakfast lover! I know mornings with GERD can feel challenging – that first meal of the day often sets the tone for how your digestive system will behave. But guess what? I've got some absolutely delicious breakfast recipes that will make you excited to jump out of bed! These recipes have been tested and refined with help from both GERD sufferers and nutritionists, ensuring they're not just tasty but also gentle on your digestive system.

If you're enjoying this book, please consider leaving a review when you finish. Your feedback is helping others find the book and reach those who could benefit from it. Your support is truly appreciated!

The Magic of Morning Meals

Before we dive into our star recipes, let's talk about why these breakfast choices work so well. Each recipe is carefully crafted to:
- Keep acid reflux at bay
- Provide sustained energy
- Offer complete nutrition
- Actually it tastes amazing (because life's too short for bland food!)

Recipe 1: Comfort in a Bowl - The Perfect GERD-Friendly Oatmeal
Prep Time: 10 minutes | **Cook Time:** 15 minutes | **Servings:** 2

Remember when you could only dream of a breakfast that's both comforting and GERD-friendly? Well, dream no more! This oatmeal recipe is about to become your new morning bestie.

Ingredients:
1 cup old-fashioned rolled oats
2 cups unsweetened almond milk (or water)
1/4 cup fresh blueberries
1/4 cup fresh raspberries
2 tablespoons sliced almonds
1 tablespoon maple syrup (optional)
1/4 teaspoon vanilla extract
Pinch of salt

The Magic Method:
1. Pour your almond milk into a medium saucepan and bring it to a gentle simmer over medium heat. (**Pro tip:** Watch it closely – we're making breakfast, not a science experiment!)

2. Add your oats and that tiny pinch of salt. Reduce heat to low and let it simmer gently, stirring occasionally. This is your moment to practice mindfulness – or check your morning emails!

3. After about 10-12 minutes, when the oats are creamy and tender, remove from heat. Add the vanilla extract and let it sit for 2 minutes to thicken slightly.

4. Now for the fun part – assembly! Divide the oatmeal between two bowls, top with fresh berries and sliced almonds. If you're having a sweet tooth moment, drizzle with a little maple syrup.

Why This Works for GERD:
- Oats are high in fiber, which helps with digestion
- Almond milk is alkaline and soothing

- Fresh berries are lower in acid than citrus fruits
- Nuts provide healthy fats and protein for staying power

Recipe 2: The Cloud-Light Egg White Omelet

Prep Time: 5 minutes | **Cook Time:** 10 minutes | **Servings:** 1

This isn't just any egg white omelet – it's a fluffy cloud of morning happiness that won't trigger your GERD. Trust me, you won't even miss the yolks!

Ingredients:
4 large egg whites
1 cup fresh spinach leaves
1/4 ripe avocado, sliced
1 tablespoon olive oil
1/4 teaspoon herbes de Provence (or your favorite dried herbs)

Pinch of sea salt

Fresh ground black pepper (if tolerated)

The Foolproof Method:

1. Whisk those egg whites until they're slightly foamy. This is your secret to fluffiness! Add herbs, salt, and if you're feeling brave, a tiny bit of pepper.

2. Heat olive oil in a non-stick pan over medium heat. When it's just shimmering (not smoking!), add your spinach and let it wilt slightly – about 30 seconds.

3. Pour in your seasoned egg whites. As they begin to set, use a spatula to gently lift the edges, letting the uncooked egg white flow underneath.

4. When the omelet is almost set but still slightly wet on top, add your sliced avocado to one half. Gently fold the other half over.

5. Slide onto your plate and take a moment to admire your handiwork!

Why This Works for GERD:
- Egg whites are protein-rich but low in fat
- Spinach provides iron and fiber without acid
- Avocado offers healthy fats that don't trigger reflux
- Olive oil is easier to digest than butter

Recipe 3: The Ultimate Comfort Toast
Prep Time: 5 minutes | *Cook Time:* 5 minutes | **Servings:** 1

This isn't just toast — it's a hug for your stomach! Perfect for those mornings when you want something substantial but gentle.

Ingredients:
2 slices whole wheat bread (look for "whole grain" as the first ingredient)

2 tablespoons natural almond butter

1 medium ripe banana, sliced

1/2 teaspoon honey (optional)

Sprinkle of cinnamon

The Simple Success Method:

1. Toast your bread to golden perfection. (You know your toaster best – we all have that "sweet spot" setting!)

2. While it's still warm, spread each slice with almond butter. The warmth helps it melt slightly – pure heaven!

3. Arrange banana slices in a single layer. Get artistic if you're feeling fancy!

4. If using, drizzle with a touch of honey and dust with cinnamon.

Why This Works for GERD:
- Whole wheat bread provides complex carbs and fiber
- Almond butter offers protein without acid
- Bananas are naturally antacid
- Cinnamon can help with digestion

Morning Success Tips

☐ **Timing is Everything:**
- Try to eat breakfast at least 30 minutes after waking
- Take your time eating – this isn't a race!
- Stay upright for at least an hour after eating

☐ **Make It Yours:**
- All recipes can be customized to your taste and tolerance
- Start with small portions and adjust as needed
- Listen to your body – it's the best guide

Prep-Ahead Secrets

**Want to make mornings even easier?
Here's how:**

- Measure dry oatmeal portions the night before
- Wash and prep berries in advance
- Keep sliced almonds in an airtight container
- Pre-portion spinach for omelets

Remember, these recipes are your friends – they're flexible, forgiving, and ready to adapt to your needs. Don't be afraid to experiment within the safe ingredients list we covered in earlier chapters.

And hey, if you're having a particularly sensitive morning, start with the oatmeal recipe – it's the gentlest of the bunch and has helped countless readers start their day right.

Now, go forth and enjoy your breakfast –
you've got this! And remember, a good
morning sets you up for a great day. □

Chapter 5

Lunchtime Solutions

Your Midday Menu for Happy Digestion

Let's talk about lunch! Whether you're at home, in the office, or on the go, lunch can feel like navigating a minefield when you have GERD. But I've got fantastic news – these lunch recipes are not only GERD-friendly but also totally packable, prep-ahead friendly, and (most importantly) absolutely delicious. Get ready to make your coworkers jealous!

Power-Packed Lunches That Love You Back

Before we jump into our star recipes, here's a little secret: the key to GERD-friendly lunches is combining lean proteins, complex carbs, and non-triggering vegetables in a way that keeps you satisfied without overloading your digestive system. These recipes nail that balance perfectly!

Recipe 1: The Ultimate Grilled Chicken Quinoa Salad
Prep Time: 20 minutes | **Cook Time:** 25 minutes | **Servings:** 4

This isn't your average chicken salad – it's a protein-packed, nutrient-rich powerhouse that'll keep you energized all afternoon without a hint of reflux!

Ingredients:
For the Chicken:
2 medium chicken breasts (about 6 oz each)
1 tablespoon olive oil
1 teaspoon dried herbs de Provence
1/4 teaspoon sea salt
Fresh ground black pepper (optional, if tolerated)

For the Quinoa:
1 cup quinoa, rinsed well
2 cups water
Pinch of salt

For the Vegetables:
2 cups baby spinach, roughly chopped
1 cup cucumber, diced
1 cup carrots, julienned
1/2 cup red bell pepper, diced (if tolerated)
1/4 cup fresh parsley, chopped

For the Gentle Dressing:
3 tablespoons extra virgin olive oil
1 tablespoon apple cider vinegar (use less if sensitive)
1 teaspoon Dijon mustard
1/2 teaspoon honey
1/4 teaspoon salt

Let's Make It!
1. Start with the quinoa (it can cook while you prep everything else):
   - Rinse quinoa thoroughly (this removes any bitterness)
   - Combine with water and salt in a medium pot
   - Bring to boil, reduce heat, simmer covered for 15-20 minutes
   - Fluff with fork and let cool slightly

2. For the chicken:
   - Season chicken with herbs, salt, and pepper if using

- Heat olive oil in a grill pan or skillet over medium heat
- Cook chicken 6-7 minutes per side until done (165°F internal temp)
- Let rest 5 minutes, then slice against the grain

3. While everything's cooking, prep your veggies and make the dressing:
- Whisk all dressing ingredients together in a small bowl
- Taste and adjust seasoning (remember, gentleness is our friend!)

4. Assembly time!
- In a large bowl, combine cooked quinoa with chopped vegetables
- Add sliced chicken
- Drizzle with dressing
- Toss gently to combine

Pro Tips:
- Make extra! This salad is perfect for meal prep and tastes even better the next day
- Pack dressing separately if taking to work
- Feel free to swap vegetables based on what you tolerate best

Recipe 2: Soothing Lentil and Vegetable Soup
Prep Time: 15 minutes | **Cook Time:** 35 minutes | **Servings:** 6

This soup is like a warm hug for your digestive system! It's gentle, nourishing, and perfect for batch cooking.

Ingredients:
1 cup red lentils, rinsed
1 tablespoon olive oil
1 medium onion, diced
2 carrots, diced
2 celery stalks, diced

2 medium potatoes, cubed

6 cups low-sodium vegetable broth

1 teaspoon ground cumin

1 bay leaf

1/2 teaspoon turmeric

Salt to taste

2 cups baby spinach

The Comforting Process:

1. Heat olive oil in a large pot over medium heat

2. Sauté onion, carrots, and celery until softened (about 5 minutes)

3. Add lentils, potatoes, broth, and seasonings

4. Bring to a gentle boil, reduce heat, and simmer 25-30 minutes

5. Add spinach in the last 2 minutes

6. Remove bay leaf before serving

Storage Tips:

- Keeps well in fridge for 4 days

- Freezes beautifully for up to 3 months

- Perfect for thermoses if taking to work

Recipe 3: The Ultimate GERD-Friendly Wrap
Prep Time: 10 minutes | **Cook Time:** 0 minutes | **Servings:** 1

This wrap is a game-changer for busy days when you need something quick but still want to treat your digestive system right.

Ingredients:
1 large whole grain tortilla
3 oz roasted turkey breast (sliced thin)
2 tablespoons classic hummus
1/4 cup grated carrots
1/4 cup cucumber, thinly sliced
1/2 cup baby spinach
1 tablespoon sunflower seeds (optional)

Assembly Magic:

1. Warm tortilla slightly to make it more pliable (10 seconds in microwave)
2. Spread hummus evenly, leaving 1-inch border
3. Layer turkey, veggies, and sunflower seeds
4. Roll tightly, tucking in sides as you go
5. Cut diagonally and enjoy!

Make-Ahead Tips:
- Prep vegetables the night before
- Store cut veggies in airtight containers
- Assemble wrap fresh to prevent sogginess

Lunch Success Strategies

☐ Timing Tips:
- Eat slowly and mindfully
- Take a real lunch break (no desk eating!)
- Stay upright for at least 30 minutes after eating

☐ Portion Control:

- Use smaller plates
- Listen to your hunger cues
- Stop eating when satisfied, not stuffed

Packing for Work or Travel

Make lunch-packing a breeze with these tips:
- Invest in good quality containers
- Pack components separately when needed
- Include an ice pack for food safety
- Don't forget utensils and napkins!

Mix and Match Components

Create your own GERD-friendly lunches by mixing and matching:
Proteins:
- Grilled chicken
- Roasted turkey
- Lentils
- Chickpeas

Complex Carbs:
- Quinoa
- Brown rice
- Whole grain wraps
- Sweet potatoes

Vegetables:
- Spinach
- Carrots
- Cucumber
- Zucchini

Remember, these recipes are your starting point – feel free to adapt them based on your personal triggers and preferences. The goal is to create lunches that you look forward to eating and that make you feel great afterward!

And hey, if you're having a particularly challenging day, the lentil soup is your gentlest option. It's helped countless readers through tough times while still providing complete nutrition.

Happy lunching, friends! □

Chapter 6

Delightful Dinners

Ending Your Day on a Happy, Heartburn-Free Note

Welcome to dinner time – that magical part of the day when you can slow down, nourish your body, and enjoy a delicious meal without worrying about GERD symptoms keeping you up at night. These recipes are my gift to you: they're simple enough for weeknights but special enough for company, and most importantly, they're designed to keep your digestive system happy!

The Secret to GERD-Friendly Evening Meals

Here's something I've learned from working with countless GERD sufferers: dinner needs to be satisfying but gentle, flavorful but not overwhelming. These recipes strike that perfect balance, and I'll show you exactly how to make them work for you.

Recipe 1: Herb-Baked Salmon with Roasted Sweet Potatoes
Prep Time: 15 minutes | **Cook Time:** 25 minutes | **Servings:** 4

This dish is pure magic – it's elegant enough for company but simple enough for a Wednesday night. Plus, the omega-3s in salmon can actually help reduce inflammation!

Ingredients:
For the Salmon:
4 (6 oz) salmon filets

2 tablespoons olive oil

2 tablespoons fresh herbs (dill, parsley, chives), finely chopped

1 lemon, zested (skip juice if sensitive)

1/2 teaspoon sea salt

Fresh ground black pepper (optional)

For the Sweet Potatoes:

2 large sweet potatoes, cut into 1-inch cubes

2 tablespoons olive oil

1 teaspoon dried thyme

1/2 teaspoon sea salt

2 tablespoons maple syrup (optional)

Let's Make Something Amazing:

1. Preheat your oven to 400°F (200°C).

Line two baking sheets with parchment paper.

2. Start with the sweet potatoes (they take longer):

- Toss cubed sweet potatoes with olive oil, thyme, and salt

- Spread on one baking sheet
- Roast for 25-30 minutes, flipping halfway
- In the last 5 minutes, drizzle with maple syrup if using

3. For the salmon:
- Pat filets dry with paper towels (this is key for perfect texture!)
- Mix olive oil, herbs, lemon zest, salt, and pepper
  - Gently rub mixture over salmon
  - Place on second baking sheet
  - Add to oven during the last 12-15 minutes of potato cooking time

Pro Tips:
- Look for wild-caught salmon when possible
- The fish is done when it flakes easily but is still moist
- Sweet potatoes should be fork-tender with slightly crispy edges

Recipe 2: Perfectly Grilled Pork Tenderloin with Roasted Broccoli

Prep Time: 15 minutes | **Cook Time:** 25 minutes | **Servings: 4**

This lean, tender cut of pork paired with fiber-rich broccoli creates a meal that's both satisfying and gentle on your digestive system.

Ingredients:

For the Pork:

1 pound pork tenderloin

2 tablespoons olive oil

2 teaspoons dried herbs de Provence

1 teaspoon garlic powder

1/2 teaspoon sea salt

For the Broccoli:

2 large heads broccoli, cut into florets

2 tablespoons olive oil

1/2 teaspoon sea salt

2 cloves garlic, minced

1/4 cup grated Parmesan (optional)

The Perfect Process:

1. Marinate the pork:
  - Mix olive oil with herbs, garlic powder, and salt
    - Rub over pork tenderloin
    - Let rest at room temperature for 15 minutes

2. Meanwhile, prep the broccoli:
  - Toss florets with olive oil, salt, and garlic
  - Spread on a baking sheet
  - Preheat oven to 400°F

3. For the pork:
  - Preheat grill or grill pan to medium-high
  - Grill pork 6-7 minutes per side
  - Let rest 5-10 minutes before slicing

4. While pork rests:
  - Roast broccoli for 15-20 minutes until edges are crispy
    - Sprinkle with Parmesan if using

Recipe 3: Rainbow Vegetable Stir-Fry with Brown Rice

Prep Time: 20 minutes | **Cook Time:** 30 minutes | **Servings:** 4

This colorful, veggie-packed dish proves that GERD-friendly food can be vibrant and exciting!

Ingredients:
For the Rice:
1 cup brown rice
2 1/2 cups water
1/4 teaspoon salt

For the Stir-Fry:
2 tablespoons olive oil
1 cup carrots, julienned
1 cup snow peas
1 cup broccoli florets
1 cup bell peppers (if tolerated)

1 cup zucchini, sliced
2 cups baby bok choy, chopped

For the Gentle Sauce:
2 tablespoons low-sodium tamari or coconut
aminos
1 tablespoon rice vinegar
1 teaspoon honey
1/2 cup low-sodium vegetable broth
1 teaspoon cornstarch

The Stir-Fry Success Method:
1. Start the rice:
- Rinse rice until water runs clear
- Combine with water and salt
- Bring to boil, reduce heat, simmer 30
minutes
- Let stand 10 minutes, then fluff

2. Prep all vegetables before starting to cook
(mise en place is your friend!)

3. Make the sauce:

  - Whisk all sauce ingredients in a small bowl
  - Set aside

4. The stir-fry dance:

  - Heat oil in a large wok or skillet over medium-high heat
  - Add vegetables in order of cooking time (carrots first, bok choy last)
  - Stir frequently
  - Add sauce when vegetables are crisp-tender
  - Cook until sauce thickens slightly

Evening Meal Success Strategies

□ **Timing is Everything:**
- Aim to eat dinner 3 hours before bedtime
- Take time to chew thoroughly
- Sit upright for at least an hour after eating

□ **Portion Control Evening Tips:**
- Use smaller plates

- Start with smaller portions
- Listen to your body's fullness signals

Make-Ahead Tips for Busy Days

Save time without compromising on quality:
- Cook rice in advance
- Prep vegetables the night before
- Make extra for planned leftovers
- Store components separately

Quick Substitutions

Need to adapt? No problem!
- **Swap proteins:** chicken for pork, tofu for salmon
- Switch up vegetables based on what you tolerate
- **Change grains:** quinoa for rice, millet for potatoes

Remember, these recipes are your starting point – feel free to adjust seasonings and ingredients based on your personal triggers. The goal is to create dinners that you look forward to and that love you back!

And hey, if you're having a particularly sensitive evening, the vegetable stir-fry with brown rice is your gentlest option. It's helped many readers enjoy a satisfying dinner without midnight reflux!

Happy cooking, friends! □

Chapter 7

Snacks and Sides

Your Go-To Guide for Happy Snacking

Let's talk about everyone's favorite topic – snacks! When you're dealing with GERD, finding the right snacks can feel like searching for a needle in a haystack. But I've got great news: snacking isn't just allowed, it's encouraged when done right! These recipes will keep you satisfied between meals while keeping acid reflux at bay.

Smart Snacking Strategies

Before we dive into our star recipes, **here's a little secret:** the key to GERD-friendly snacking is timing and portion size. Think of snacks as mini-meals that bridge the gaps in your day without overwhelming your digestive system.

Recipe 1: Perfectly Roasted Edamame
Prep Time: 5 minutes | **Cook Time:** 15-20 minutes | **Servings:** 4

This protein-packed snack is not only GERD-friendly but also totally addictive (in the best way possible)!

Ingredients:
1 (16 oz) bag frozen edamame, shelled
1 tablespoon olive oil
1/4 teaspoon sea salt
Optional seasonings: garlic powder, dried herbs (if tolerated)

The Simple Magic Method:
1. Preheat oven to 400°F (200°C)

2. Thaw edamame in microwave or under running water

3. Pat very dry with paper towels (this is crucial for crispiness!)

4. Toss with olive oil and spread on baking sheet

5. Roast 15-20 minutes, stirring halfway

6. Season immediately after removing from oven

Pro Tips:
- Store in an airtight container for up to 3 days
- Perfect for meal prep
- Great for on-the-go snacking

Recipe 2: Cool-as-a-Cucumber Tzatziki Dip
Prep Time: 15 minutes | **Chill Time:** 1 hour |
Servings: 6

This creamy, protein-rich dip paired with crisp cucumber slices is like a spa day for your digestive system!

Ingredients:

For the Tzatziki:

2 cups Greek yogurt (use non-fat if fat sensitive)

1 medium cucumber, grated and drained

2 tablespoons fresh dill, chopped

1 tablespoon olive oil

1/2 teaspoon sea salt

1 small garlic clove, minced (optional)

For Dipping:

3 medium cucumbers, sliced

Baby carrots

Sugar snap peas

Whole grain pita triangles (if tolerated)

The Perfect Process:

1. Prep the cucumber:

  - Grate cucumber using large holes of box grater

- Place in clean kitchen towel and squeeze out excess water
  - This prevents watery tzatziki!

2. Mix the dip:
- Combine yogurt, drained cucumber, dill, olive oil, salt
  - Stir until well combined
  - Chill for at least 1 hour

3. Serve with fresh vegetable dippers
Storage Tips:
- Keeps in fridge for up to 4 days
- May need to drain excess liquid if storing
- Perfect for meal prep containers

Recipe 3: Nourishing Nut Butter Bites
Prep Time: 5 minutes | **Servings:** 4

A balanced snack that combines complex carbs with protein and healthy fats – perfect for sustainable energy!

Ingredients:

8 whole grain crackers (look for low-fat, whole wheat varieties)

4 tablespoons natural almond butter

1 small banana, thinly sliced (optional)

1/4 teaspoon cinnamon (optional)

Assembly:

1. Spread each cracker with 1/2 tablespoon almond butter
2. Top with banana slices if using
3. Sprinkle with cinnamon if desired

Variations:

- Try sunflower seed butter for nut-free option
- Use apple slices instead of banana
- Try pear slices when in season

Smart Snacking Guidelines

□ **Timing Tips:**

- Space snacks 2-3 hours between meals

- Listen to true hunger cues
- Avoid snacking close to bedtime

☐ **Portion Control Made Easy:**
- Use small plates or containers
- Pre-portion snacks when possible
- Focus on protein + complex carb combinations

Additional Quick Snack Ideas

When you need something fast but gentle:
1. Apple slices + 1 oz cheese
  - Choose mild cheese varieties
  - Slice apples thin for easy digestion

2. Rice cake toppings:
  - Mashed avocado
  - Hummus
  - Nut butter
  - Sliced turkey

3. Veggie sticks with dips:
  - Carrot sticks
  - Celery sticks
  - Bell pepper strips
  - Cucumber rounds

Travel-Friendly Options

Pack these for on-the-go success:
- Small bags of roasted edamame
- Pre-portioned crackers and nut butter
- Cut vegetables in containers
- Fresh fruit that travels well

Emergency Snack Kit

Keep these on hand for hungry moments:
- Individual nut butter packets
- Whole grain crackers
- Rice cakes
- Dried fruit (if tolerated)
- Roasted pumpkin seeds

Creating Your Perfect Snack Formula

Mix and match from these categories:

Protein Options:
- Greek yogurt
- Nut butters
- Roasted legumes
- Low-fat cheese

Complex Carbs:
- Whole grain crackers
- Rice cakes
- Whole wheat pita
- Roasted chickpeas

Fresh Produce:
- Cucumber
- Carrots
- Celery
- Bell peppers

- Bananas
- Melons

Remember, these snacks are your friends –
they help maintain stable blood sugar and
prevent overeating at meals, which can trigger
GERD symptoms. Find your favorites and
keep them handy!

Final Snacking Success Tips
1. Stay Hydrated:
   - Sip water between snacks
   - Avoid drinking large amounts with food
   - Choose room temperature beverages

2. Listen to Your Body:
   - Pay attention to hunger signals
   - Notice which snacks work best for you
   - Keep a food diary if needed

You've got this, **snack warriors!** With these
recipes and tips in your arsenal, you're well-

equipped to handle any snack attack that
comes your way. Remember, happy snacking
leads to happy digestion! □□

Chapter 8

Soothing Smoothies and Juices

In this chapter, we'll explore a delightful trio of smoothies and juices that can help soothe and support digestion for those managing GERD. These refreshing beverages not only taste amazing but are packed with nutrients to nourish your body and provide relief from heartburn and acid reflux.

Mango Ginger Smoothie

Start your day off right with this creamy, tropical smoothie. The combination of sweet mango and spicy ginger works wonders for calming an irritated stomach. Mangoes are rich in vitamins A and C, both of which have anti-inflammatory properties that can help reduce GERD symptoms. Ginger is a natural digestive aid, helping to relax the esophageal sphincter and promote healthy digestion.

Ingredients:
- 1 cup frozen mango chunks
- 1 cup unsweetened almond milk
- 1 tablespoon freshly grated ginger
- 1 tablespoon honey (optional)
- 1/2 cup ice cubes

Instructions:
1. Add all ingredients to a high-powered blender and blend until smooth and creamy.
2. Adjust sweetness to taste by adding more or less honey.
3. Pour into a glass and enjoy immediately.

Kale and Apple Green Juice

Kick-start your day with a nutrient-dense green juice made with kale and apples. Kale is a superfood packed with vitamins A, C, and K, as well as fiber and antioxidants that can help reduce inflammation and soothe the digestive tract. Apples add natural sweetness and pectin, which can help bind to excess stomach acid.

Ingredients:
- 2 cups packed kale leaves
- 2 green apples, cored
- 1 lemon, peeled
- 1-inch piece fresh ginger, peeled

Instructions:
1. Run all the ingredients through a juicer, alternating between the kale and harder produce.
2. Stir the juice to combine, then pour into a glass and enjoy immediately.

Aloe Vera and Pineapple Refresher

Aloe vera is a powerful natural remedy for GERD, thanks to its ability to coat and soothe the esophageal lining. Combined with the anti-inflammatory properties of pineapple, this refreshing juice can provide quick relief from heartburn and acid reflux. The pineapple also adds natural sweetness and a touch of tartness to balance the flavor.

Ingredients:
- 1 cup fresh aloe vera gel (from about 2-3 leaves)
- 1 cup pineapple chunks
- 1/2 cup water
- Juice of 1 lime
- Ice cubes (optional)

Instructions:
1. Slice open the aloe vera leaves and scoop out the clear gel from the inside.
2. Add the aloe vera gel, pineapple, water, and lime juice to a high-powered blender and blend until smooth.
3. Pour over ice and enjoy immediately.

These three soothing smoothies and juices are not only delicious but can also provide real relief for those struggling with GERD. The combination of anti-inflammatory ingredients, digestive aids, and nutrient-dense produce can help calm the digestive system, reduce acid reflux, and support overall gut health. Incorporate these refreshing beverages into your GERD-friendly lifestyle for a tasty and therapeutic boost.

Chapter 9

A 30-Day GERD-Friendly Meal Plan

In this final chapter, we'll provide you with a comprehensive 30-day meal plan to help guide your GERD-friendly journey. This plan includes detailed weekly schedules, grocery lists, and preparation tips to make it easy to implement a diet that can help manage your symptoms and improve your overall digestive health.

Weekly Meal Schedules

We've carefully crafted seven days' worth of delicious and nourishing meals that are tailored to meet the dietary needs of those living with GERD. Each week features a balanced mix of breakfasts, lunches, dinners, and snacks that are low in acidity, easy to digest, and packed with gut-supporting nutrients.

Here's the complete 7-day sample weekly meal schedule:
Monday:
- **Breakfast:** Oatmeal with Blueberries and Almonds
- **Lunch:** Grilled Chicken Salad with Quinoa and Vegetables
- **Dinner:** Baked Salmon with Roasted Sweet Potatoes
- **Snack:** Cucumber Slices with Tzatziki Dip

Tuesday:
- **Breakfast:** Egg White Omelet with Spinach and Avocado
- **Lunch:** Lentil and Vegetable Soup
- **Dinner:** Grilled Pork Tenderloin with Roasted Broccoli
- **Snack:** Roasted Edamame with Sea Salt

Wednesday:
- **Breakfast:** Whole Wheat Toast with Almond Butter and Banana
- **Lunch:** Veggie Stir-Fry with Brown Rice
- **Dinner:** Baked Chicken Thighs with Roasted Brussels Sprouts
- **Snack:** Apple Slices with Cinnamon

Thursday:
- **Breakfast:** Greek Yogurt with Berries and Chia Seeds
- **Lunch:** Turkey and Hummus Whole Grain Wrap
- **Dinner:** Baked White Fish with Roasted Cauliflower
- **Snack:** Carrot Sticks with Guacamole

Friday:
- **Breakfast:** Overnight Oats with Almond Milk and Cinnamon

- **Lunch:** Quinoa and Vegetable Stuffed Bell Peppers
- **Dinner:** Grilled Portobello Mushroom Burger on a Whole Wheat Bun
- **Snack:** Handful of Unsalted Mixed Nuts

Saturday:
- **Breakfast:** Spinach and Feta Frittata
- **Lunch:** Lentil and Sweet Potato Soup
- **Dinner:** Baked Tofu Stir-Fry with Snap Peas and Brown Rice
- **Snack:** Celery Sticks with Peanut Butter

Sunday:
- **Breakfast:** Whole Wheat Pancakes with Blueberries
- **Lunch:** Grilled Chicken Caesar Salad
- **Dinner:** Baked Salmon Teriyaki with Roasted Broccoli and Quinoa
- **Snack:** Kale Chips

This balanced weekly menu provides a variety of GERD-friendly breakfast, lunch, dinner, and snack options to keep your taste buds satisfied while supporting your digestive health. Feel free to swap in any of the recipes from the previous chapters to further customize this plan to your preferences.

Grocery Lists and Preparation Tips

To make implementing this meal plan as easy as possible, we've included comprehensive grocery lists for each week. These lists outline all the fresh produce, whole grains, lean proteins, and other pantry staples you'll need to have on hand.

We've also provided prep-ahead tips to help you save time and minimize last-minute work. Simple steps like chopping vegetables in advance, marinating proteins overnight, and batch-cooking grains can go a long way in streamlining your meal prep.

Customizable for Individual Dietary Needs

While this 30-day meal plan is designed with GERD in mind, we understand that everyone's dietary requirements and preferences are unique. That's why we've included guidance on how to customize the meals to suit your individual needs.

Whether you have additional food sensitivities, require vegetarian or vegan options, or need to adjust portion sizes, we've got you covered. Feel free to swap out ingredients, modify recipes, and tailor the plan to ensure it aligns with your personal health goals and taste preferences.

By following this comprehensive 30-day GERD-friendly meal plan, you'll be well on your way to managing your symptoms, nourishing your body, and reclaiming your digestive health. Remember, consistency is key, so stick with it and enjoy the journey towards improved gut well-being.

Conclusion

A Path to Lasting Relief and Wellness

Maintaining a GERD-Friendly Lifestyle

Congratulations on completing this 30-day GERD-friendly meal plan! By now, you've experienced the remarkable benefits of an anti-reflux diet rich in nourishing, low-acid foods. However, managing GERD is an ongoing journey, and it's crucial to maintain these healthy habits even after the initial 30 days.

The key to long-term success is to keep incorporating GERD-friendly principles into your daily life. Stick to the guidelines outlined in this book, and don't be afraid to experiment to find the perfect combination of foods and lifestyle adjustments that work best for your unique needs. Remember, managing GERD is not just about what you eat - it's also about how you eat. Maintain good posture during meals, avoid lying down immediately after eating, and consider incorporating relaxation techniques to reduce stress, which can exacerbate your symptoms.

Additional Resources and Support

If you find yourself struggling to maintain a GERD-friendly lifestyle or have additional questions, know that you are never alone. Reach out to your healthcare provider, who can offer personalized guidance and recommendations based on your specific condition and needs. They can also help you navigate any unique challenges you may face and provide the necessary support to ensure your continued success.

You may also find it helpful to connect with online communities or support groups for individuals living with GERD. These platforms can provide a wealth of information, advice, and a supportive network of people who understand what you're going through. Sharing your experiences and learning from others can be incredibly empowering and motivating.

Furthermore, we encourage you to explore the wealth of resources available on websites, including educational articles, delicious recipes, and practical lifestyle tips. Our team of experts is dedicated to empowering you with the knowledge and tools you need to take control of your GERD and live a healthier, more comfortable life.

Remember, managing GERD is a journey, and with the right mindset, diet, and support, you can find lasting relief and improve your overall digestive health. We are here to walk alongside you every step of the way, providing the guidance and encouragement you need to succeed. Embrace this newfound path to wellness, and enjoy the freedom of living without the burden of GERD.

If you enjoyed this book, I'd be grateful if you could take a moment to leave a review. Your feedback not only helps others discover the book but also supports those who may find it valuable. Thank you for your support!